Two Feet
from our Thoughts

by

Adrian M. Seager

First edition published in the UK, 2000
© Adrian M. Seager

32 Priory Road
Portbury
Bristol
BS20 7TH

Typeset by Copyprint, Portishead, North Somerset
Author's photograph by Mitchell Duncan & Associates Ltd.
Book cover Westspring Graphics

ISBN No: 0-9537832-0-0

"Two Feet from our Thoughts"

CONTENTS

ACKNOWLEDGEMENTS

Thanks are accorded to Dr. Barry Durrant-Peatfield for his interest and for his kindness in writing the Foreword to this little book. Also, to Nigel Vukovich for kindly allowing me to base the section on leg ulcers upon notes gleaned at one of his very informative seminars some years ago.

I am indebted to the SMAE Institute for its quality, theoretical and practical training in surgical chiropody and to the International Institute of Reflexology for opening the door to a new life.

No work of this nature is possible without the help and support of our nearest and dearest and it is thanks to my wife, Norma, for that and for proof-reading the material.

I would also like to thank Amanda and Mike Sanders of 'Printacopy' for their invaluable advice and guidance during the compilation of the book - we have even studied the reader's eyesight in choosing a clear typeface that we trust you find easy to read.

Finally, a great debt of gratitude to my Secretary, Gill, for her tolerance, patience and good ideas throughout, not least for the production of the draft from which the printers were able to produce this book.

FOREWORD

by

Dr. Barry J. Durrant-Peatfield
MD, BS, LRCP, MRCS, CAM

As Adrian Seager correctly notes, we do rather take our feet for granted. Disorders of the feet can quite ruin people's lives and cause endless and unremitting pain. Not only is it true that the average person does not think about their feet, but I am sorry to say that we doctors don't either.

Or at least we didn't. I have read Adrian's clear, lucid and accurate account of feet and their problems with huge interest. I am amazed that there was so much to learn; but absorb it I have, and am much wiser for it. As a doctor who greatly values the work of reflexologists, with particular knowledge of Adrian's work, I found my perspectives enlarging and my understanding growing. So also will you, the reader.

I would wish every doctor to read, enjoy and learn from this book, as I have done; and I would wish it to be included in every medical student's curriculum.

Barry J. Durrant-Peatfield
The Foxley Lane Clinic Limited

INTRODUCTION

Have you given a thought to your feet today? Of course not, you probably sat on the bed, thrust them into your slippers or shoes and expected them to function long before your others parts awoke.

Yet, the expansion of the chiropody profession is testimony to an increasing number of people suffering pain, discomfort or disability of the feet and lower limbs.

Shoes that are well designed and fitted can do much to alleviate these problems.

However, it is more likely that few of us have stopped to think what the foot is expected to endure.

Imagine, for a moment, the average adult walking stride of about one metre, during which the foot impacts, bends, stretches and twists under our body weight. This occurs about a thousand times for each mile we walk throughout our entire lives!

If we average two miles per day - which is a conservative figure for any housewife - that is over 700 miles every year. By the time we reach our late forties, we would have clocked up over 35,000 miles!

We don't expect our car to do this without regular servicing and **it can be replaced**. Yet, we expect it of our feet, and **they cannot be replaced** (other than by mechanical substitution).

In addition, they must bear our body weight such that, for a 10 stone person, each foot supports 70lb, when standing, and when running this force is doubled by the impact effect, and for the split second that the heel strikes the ground, this force is very much greater still. So, it is quite illogical and decidedly unfair to expect our feet to withstand this pounding and consequent wear and tear without any form of maintenance treatment.

Social Habits

Before we get too serious, however, let us consider a few social habits and values, in   relation to our attitude to foot-care.

Ladies will happily spend £20 and more on a hair cut, shampoo, set, or whatever. They spend £100 and more on an evening dress that, they tell us, has a very limited use.

Equally, men spend £40 to watch their local team, in comfort, with no guarantee of the quality of the performance; spend £10 plus on a few drinks with the lads; £40/£50 approximately for a new tyre for the car, and so on.

If the television, fridge or video-recorder breaks down it is a major domestic crisis to which the response is 'to afford' £350 - £1,000 on an instant replacement.

Yet, we are reluctant to spend, say £15 to £30, for professional treatment of our feet. This does seem a peculiar set of values!

So, This is for You

Together, the previous comments and observations became a personal and compelling reason to write a small, simple book to break the mould of complacency that leads us to take our feet for granted. We rarely give them a thought, hence the title of this book.

Primarily, it is written for any complementary therapist whose work includes the feet - particularly reflexologists. Also, it is for physiotherapists, osteopaths, chiropractors, sports injury therapists and for members of the public's general curiosity.

It does not set out to be comprehensive but to be an easy read, memory jogger and reference. For those who would like to gain a more detailed knowledge, please refer to the 'Further Reading' list at the back of this book.

Your suggestions and comments are welcome. Meanwhile, I hope it provides an enjoyable and interesting read.

Adrian M. Seager

CHAPTER I

ANATOMY OF THE FEET & TERMINOLOGY

To understand the prevention and treatment of foot ailments, requires a basic knowledge of the anatomy of the foot.

There are 26 bones in the foot (see Figure 1).

These bones are in 3 main sections (Figure 2):

- Tarsus
- Metatarsus
- Phalanges

Tarsus (Ref. Fig. 2)

Consists of:

- the largest bone in the foot, the heel bone or **calcaneum**;
- the instep bone, or **navicular**, at the top of the transverse and longitudinal arches, which is similar to the keystone in an archway;
- the **talus** bone sits on top of the dorsal facet of the calcaneum and articulates with the malleoli of the tibia and fibula to form the **ankle joint**;
- the **cuneiform bones, medial, middle and lateral**, and the **cuboid** bone completes the seven bones of the tarsus. The cuboid lies at the outer (lateral) border of the foot and anterior to a facet of the calcaneum.

Metatarsus (Ref. Fig. 2)

This section comprises the five metatarsal bones, numbered from one (at the medial, or inner border of the foot) to five. These bones, together, form the medial longitudinal arch and the lateral longitudinal arch of the foot. Their heads articulate with the corresponding heads of the toe-bones, phalanges.

Phalanges (Toes) (Ref. Fig. 2)

There are 14 bones in total: two forming the big toe, or hallux, and three in each of the other toes, numbered two to five, inclusive - where toe 5 is the smallest toe.

Muscles and Ligaments (Ref. Figs. 5 & 6)

Muscles and ligaments hold the bones in place, whilst allowing the various bones to slide, one with another - giving the necessary mobility of the foot - like a four-way sprung structure. Notice how, when elderly people lose this mobility through lack of exercise, osteoporosis, injury, illness, arthritis, neglect or abuse of the feet, they shuffle. They use their feet like sledges and, in addition, may rock the pelvis from side-to-side, like a 'Kelly'.

The Four Arches of the Foot (Ref. Figs. 3 & 4)

Medial Longitudinal Arch stretches from the medial, anterior, aspect of the **calcaneum** forward to the head of the **first metatarsal** bone: the arch consists, therefore, of the calcaneum, talus, navicular and medial cuneiform bones.

Lateral Longitudinal Arch similarly stretches from the lateral, anterior, facet of the **calcaneum** to the head of the **fifth metatarsal** bone: it consists of the cuboid and fifth metatarsal (Figure 3).

Transverse Arch is formed by the cuboid and the cuneiform bones; it extends from the lateral border or the **cuboid** across the foot to the medial facet of the **medial cuneiform** bone (Figure 2).

The Forward or Metatarsal Arch is a very important arch from which the foot derives a great deal of its suppleness and 'spring'.   Deformity of this arch can be both painful and partially immobilising. This arch stretches from the head of the **first metatarsal** bone, across the foot via the other metatarsal heads, to the **fifth metatarsal**. In a healthy foot, it forms a shallow, bowed arch across the under, plantar, surface of the forward portion of the foot - a little posterior to where the toes join the foot (Figure 2).

Function of these Arches is to provide a four-way sprung structure of the foot, so that it can flex under our body weight and thus respond to the numerous and varied load demands we place upon our feet (Figure 4).

It is important to realise that improper or poorly fitted footwear can weaken these arches.

The Attachment of the Foot to the Leg

The ankle is a simple hinge in one plane only, that is in the same line as the length of the foot. The 'pin' of the hinge is the talus bone that swivels between the distal, medial malleolus of the tibia (thick medial bone) and the distal, lateral malleolus of the fibula (thin lateral bone).

The only thing preventing this structure from falling apart are the ligaments and tendons that are wrapped around the joint and secure it whilst allowing sufficient local mobility. (Figures 5a and 5b show some of these ligaments in diagrammatic form.)

Figure 6 shows how the ligaments wrap around the bones and tendons of the foot and lower leg, rather like nature's bandages, to hold the whole structure in place.

Figure 7 shows a particular tendon on the plantar surface of the foot that has particular significance for reflexologists.

Terminology

In each step that we take there are:

- inward twisting, or **pronation**
- outward twisting, or **supination**
- bending of the top of the foot, **dorsiflexion**, and
- curving of the bottom of the foot, **plantarflexion.**

Figures 8 and 9 illustrate these terms and are intended to avoid the frequent confusion that occurs.

Similarly, it helps to appreciate that **abduction** means 'to take away from' and **adduction** means 'to add to'. Generally, these terms are used to describe movement in relation to an imaginary line through the centre of our body.

Referring to the foot and looking vertically, the centre-line of the foot is taken to be a line passing through the centre of the second toe (Figure 10). So, for a big toe that turns towards the second toe, it is said to **adduct** with reference to the foot; whilst in relation to the body as a whole, it **abducts.** Provided we are clear about whether we are referring to the whole body or just the feet, confusion can be avoided.

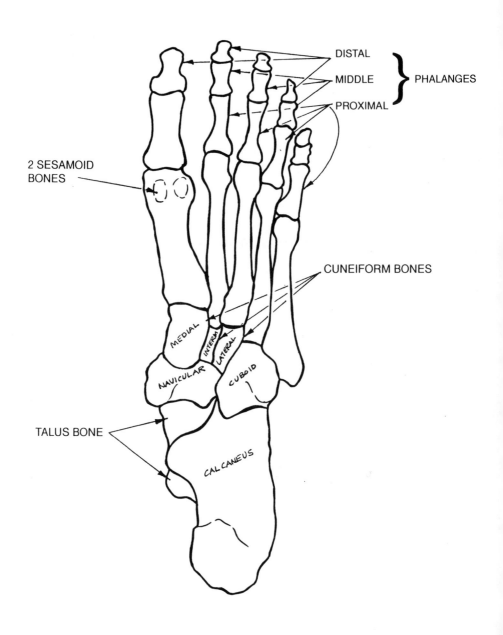

FIG 1: LEFT FOOT - PLANTAR VIEW

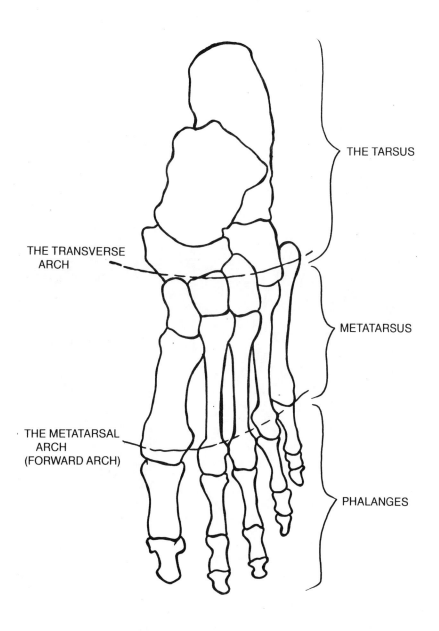

THE TARSUS

THE TRANSVERSE
ARCH

METATARSUS

THE METATARSAL
ARCH
(FORWARD ARCH)

PHALANGES

<u>FIG 2: LEFT FOOT - DORSAL VIEW</u>

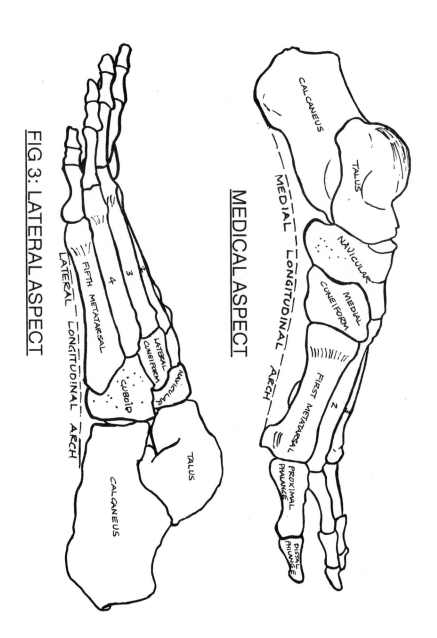

FIG 3: LATERAL ASPECT

MEDICAL ASPECT

LATERAL LONGITUDINAL ARCH

FIFTH METATARSAL

4

3

LATERAL CUNEIFORM

CUBOID

NAVICULAR

CALCANEUS

TALUS

MEDIAL LONGITUDINAL ARCH

CALCANEUS

TALUS

NAVICULAR

MEDIAL CUNEIFORM

FIRST METATARSAL

2

PROXIMAL PHALANGE

DISTALE PHALANGE

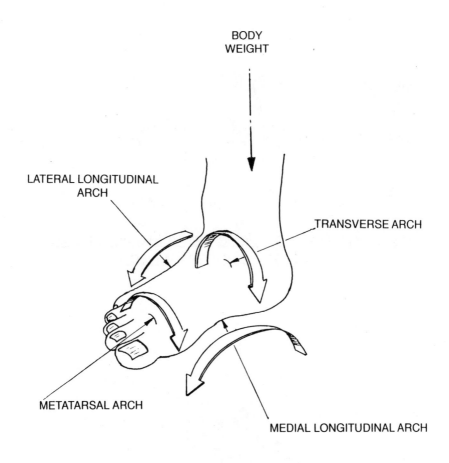

BODY
WEIGHT

LATERAL LONGITUDINAL
ARCH

TRANSVERSE ARCH

METATARSAL ARCH

MEDIAL LONGITUDINAL ARCH

FIG 4: THE FOOT AS A SPRUNG STRUCTURE
SUPPORTING THE BODY'S WEIGHT

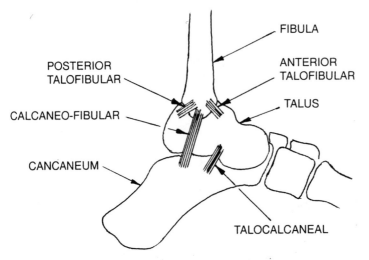

FIG 5a: SHOWING SOME OF THE LIGAMENTS THAT HOLD THE ANKLE
JOINT TOGETHER (LATERAL ASPECT)

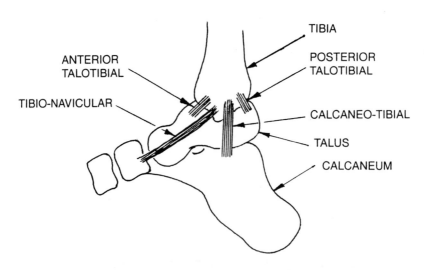

FIG 5b: SHOWING SOME OF THE MEDIAL LIGAMENTS THAT HOLD THE
ANKLE JOINT TOGETHER

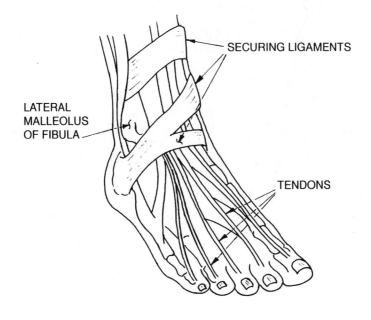

SECURING LIGAMENTS

**LATERAL
MALLEOLUS
OF FIBULA**

TENDONS

FIG 6: SKETCH SHOWING HOW LIGAMENTS ACT LIKE 'BANDAGES' TO HOLD THE ANKLE JOINT IN PLACE

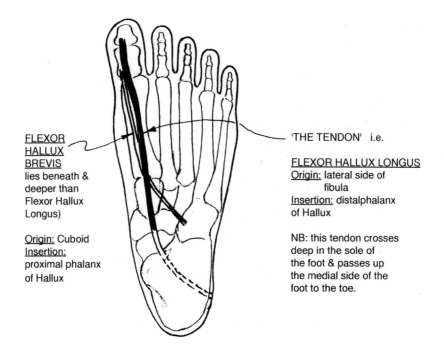

FLEXOR
HALLUX
BREVIS
lies beneath &
deeper than
Flexor Hallux
Longus)

Origin: Cuboid
Insertion:
proximal phalanx
of Hallux

'THE TENDON' i.e.

FLEXOR HALLUX LONGUS
Origin: lateral side of
          fibula
Insertion: distalphalanx
of Hallux

NB: this tendon crosses
deep in the sole of
the foot & passes up
the medial side of the
foot to the toe.

FIG 7:
SKETCH OF THE PLANTAR VIEW
OF THE LEFT FOOT
SHOWING 'THE TENDON LINE'
USED IN REFLEXOLOGY

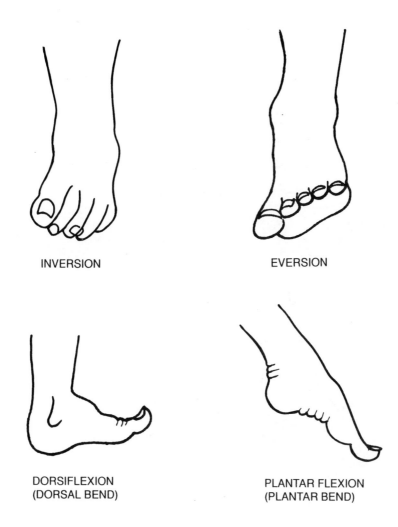

INVERSION

EVERSION

DORSIFLEXION
(DORSAL BEND)

PLANTAR FLEXION
(PLANTAR BEND)

FIG 8: TERMINOLOGY

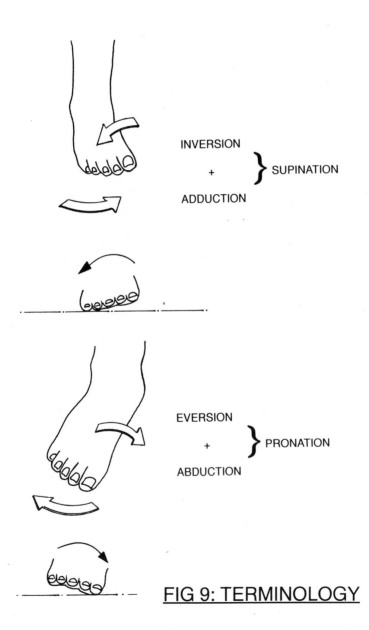

INVERSION
+
ADDUCTION
} SUPINATION

EVERSION
+
ABDUCTION
} PRONATION

FIG 9: TERMINOLOGY

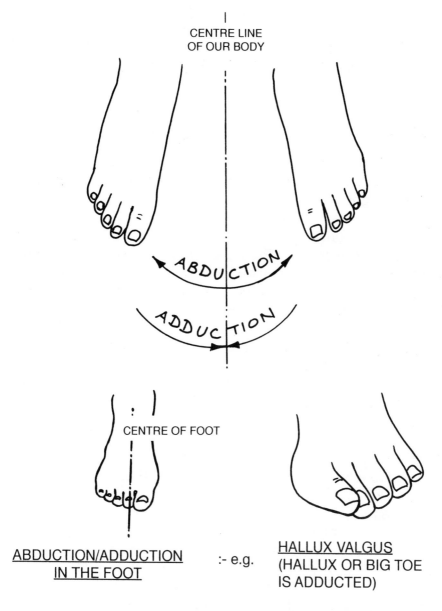

CENTRE LINE
OF OUR BODY

ABDUCTION

ADDUCTION

CENTRE OF FOOT

**ABDUCTION/ADDUCTION
IN THE FOOT**

:- e.g.

HALLUX VALGUS
(HALLUX OR BIG TOE
IS ADDUCTED)

FIG 10: TERMINOLOGY

Chapter II

Action of the Feet & Lower Limbs

Action of the Foot

When walking correctly, our heel strikes the ground squarely and, simultaneous with forward motion and consequent shift of body-weight, the foot 'rolls' from supination to pronation, i.e. from the heel-strike biased to the outside of the foot to the weight 'rolling' onto the inside of the heel in a split second of time. This is shown by Figure 8. In other words, the body weight transfers forward along the outer portion of the heel and almost immediately along the outer part of the foot. As the weight approaches the forward arch (metatarsal arch), the foot rolls inwards (adducts) and begins to bend (dorsiflexes) and pushes off via the toes, with the final and influential thrust coming from the big toe (hallux). See also Figure 11. It is a smooth, continuous movement that becomes subconscious from the time we are quite young. We don't think about it, we just do it.

Have you ever met anyone who was **taught** to walk correctly? If you have, please send me their name and address because I would like to meet that pioneer. The greatest possibility is that we all copied our closest relative or companion. Notice how often the children walk in a similar style to their parents. Sons often copy their father - or some other hero Figure, it was John Wayne or Gary Cooper in my day and Clint Eastwood in my sons' era! Whilst daughters frequently walk like their mother, whilst talking non-stop! This all leads to a fair number of the population copying faults which, over a period of years, may cause a foot-problem.

A sub normal gait and foot-structure can be involved in low back pain or pain in the hip, knee or pelvic area (often at the sacro-iliac joint). Some abnormalities can be small and, as a consequence, tolerated for many years by the sufferers. But the cumulative effect can have an adverse effect upon health generally. For example, a low back displacement can be a cause of constipation - although that condition can have other contributory factors.

Another familiar outcome of abnormal foot movement and gait is stiffness of the joints that can be progressive with age. Notice how the 'foot-sledging' of older people is a feature of their 'elderliness'. The feet do not bend, the head, neck and upper back bends to compensate: this, in turn, restricts full breathing and, together, can accelerate general degeneration of the person.

Now that you are thoroughly depressed we will attempt to cheer you up with a look at the basic foot and lower limb movements. When we understand, we are in a better position to take avoiding or corrective action that can make life more pleasant.

Our first requirement may come as a surprise. Quite simply, it is energy - the energy required to power our nervous system that signals to our muscles to contract in a sequential pattern that produces walking. When we are ill in bed, there is little or no inclination or energy for movement; all the body's energy is consumed in battling against the illness.

We possess two forms of energy. One is when we are stationary; the energy is stored and there is the potential for movement - this is called potential energy. The other form of energy is that of movement - this is called kinetic energy.

The body is constantly interchanging these two basic types of energy every time we move our limbs or trunk from static to motion, the conversion occurring without us being conscious of the process.

Impact Upon Foot & Lower Limb

Frequently, it is not appreciated that the impact of the foot on a non-giving surface transfers all the way up the lower body to the base region of the spine (coccyx, sacrum and lumbar). The impact transfers a force up through the bones below the knee-joint (the tibia and fibula) to the knee.

The knee joint consists of the heads (upper condyles) of the tibia and fibula and the lower condyle of the thigh bone (femur). To stop these bones grinding together - which would be agony - there is a cushion of cartilage that is, in turn, lubricated by a fluid called synovial fluid. Various short, very strong, ligaments criss-cross the joint which binds it together and stabilises it laterally. In addition the joint is protected at the front by a sliding cap of bone called the knee-cap or patella. This too is held in place by local ligaments.

From the knee-joint, the force of impact travels on up through the thigh bone (femur), the head of femur and into the pelvic girdle, via the acetabulum. The force is transferred up into the spine - particularly the sacrum and lumbar regions.

Understanding this transfer of force and the path it takes helps us to realise that a foot problem may lead, in time, to a back problem. This can be a displacement, rotation or misalignment with consequent pain that can, in some instances, become severe and be incapacitating. Equally, the reverse can happen, where a spinal misalignment can, in turn, cause a pain in the foot.

The necessary realisation is the connection between the apparent extremes of foot to spine and vice versa. Therefore, care and thoroughness is needed in diagnosing cause and effect. This is done best by a qualified osteopath, or by a qualified chiropractor, either by direct individual appointment or in liaison with a General Practitioner or, increasingly, by a GP referral to one of these specialist therapists.

Muscular Activity - Normal Gait

This is explained most easily by reference to Figure 11. For simplicity, we look at the right leg only. The cycle starts with all the body-weight on the left leg which allows the right leg to swing freely as the weight is moved laterally onto the left leg. The muscle at the front of the shin (tibialus anterior) contracts almost simultaneously with the muscles at the front of the thigh (quadriceps) and the one at the back of the thigh ('hamstrings' - semitendinosus, semimembranosus and bi-ceps femoris) together with the gluteus muscles, i.e. the right 'buttock' muscles.

This group of muscles acting in unison contract to allow the heel to strike the walking surface. Immediately following the heel-strike, the tibialus posterior begins to contract - to cause the heel to lift off the surface ('HO' on Figure 11) until the tibialus anterior and quadriceps again contract to lift the toe off for the start of the repeat cycle.

We never give a thought (hence the title of the book) to the fact that this sequence occurs thousands of times during our active life as our body weight and centre of gravity also move. Furthermore, the whole weight-bearing impact is increased by three times and much more (for very minute periods of time) when we jog or run. Hence too much jogging - particularly on hard, unyielding surfaces, is not good for us. Why copy the

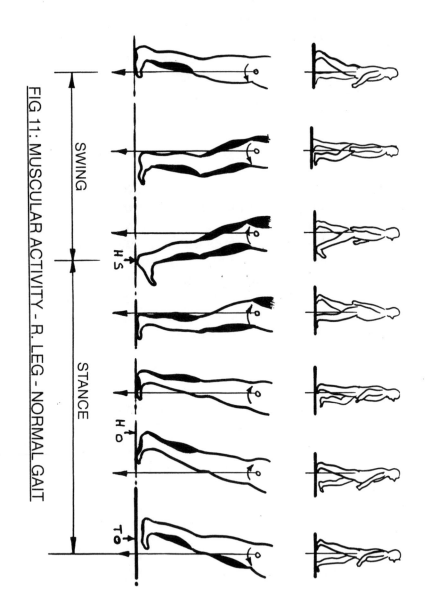

FIG 11: MUSCULAR ACTIVITY - R. LEG - NORMAL GAIT

Americans all the time? Too many of them are overweight anyway and jogging has become a fad and, in my opinion, can even become addictive. Try eating less of everything and thinking about jogging whilst resting in your favourite chair! Then go for a brisk walk or go for a swim - it does just as much good and without the harmful side effects of jarring our joints.

Chapter III

Feet as Circulation 'Pumps'

The foot not only has a great influence upon our comfort and mobility but also plays a very important part in our vascular system.

Pathologically, the veins of the sole of the foot for many years were regarded as insignificant. Anatomically, only the medial and lateral arches of the foot had received attention.

Until the work of Dr. A.M.N. Gardner, DM, MCh, FRCS and Dr. R.H. Fox, FRCR, little interest had been shown in the venous anatomy of the foot. They contributed greatly to our knowledge of the way in which blood returns from the human foot to the abdominal region, against gravitational influence.

The advent of videophlebography, non-irritant radiographic contrast media and of doppler blood-flow measuring techniques provided the means of studying the action of the foot and lower limb. This was undertaken by Drs. Fox and Gardner at the Department of Surgery and Radiology, Torbay District Hospital, Devon, in the mid 1980s'.

Initially, the focus of attention was upon the inferior vena cava because caval clips had been used previously on that vein during surgery, to prevent a pulmonary embolism. But the study widened to reveal a number of various 'pumps' of the lower limb (Figures 12a and 12b). Notice that those in the foot are on the plantar lateral part of the foot, i.e. they get temporarily flattened under body weight many times during the normal gait.

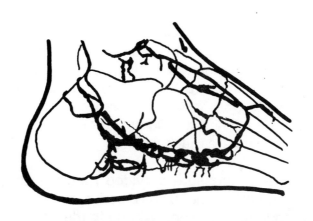

FIG 12a: NON -WEIGHTBEARING FOOT ~ FILLING OF DEEP
& SUPERFICIAL VEINS BY RADIA - OPAQUE DYE
(PHLEBOGRAM)

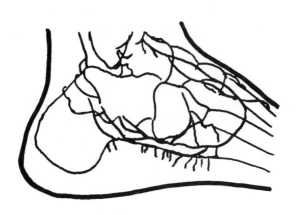

FIG 12b: WEIGHTBEARING FOOT SHOWING SUBSEQUENT
EMPTYING OF PLANTAR VEINS

FROM: BECKET & WALL, NURSING TIMES, VOL.84, NO. 19, 1988

It is this flattening, followed by expansion as the body weight is released that produces the 'pump' effect of these veins of the foot. From here the blood empties primarily up and into the anterior and posterior tibial veins: it also returns up the long and the short saphenous veins. These particular veins (the saphenous veins) are unusual in that they act as high pressure conduits (the 'foot-pump' can overcome a cuff-on-the-calf pressure inflated to 100mm of mercury). Most other subcutaneous veins are much weaker.

With the degree of pressure provided from the action of this natural 'foot-pump', a column of blood can be dislocated up beyond the abdominal region, right up to the heart.

Previously, it was believed that the plantar veins emptied only up into the dorsum of the foot.

It has been noted that the 'pump' is independent of muscular contraction since it has been observed to work well in para-plegics.

A less powerful venous 'pump' is due to the compressive action of the arterial pulse on veins enclosed within vascular bundles. The use of doppler has enabled the action to be demonstrated also in the femoral veins of paraplegics when they are in a standing position.

Videophlebography was used in Torbay Hospital from 1983, coincident with Drs. Fox and Gardner's study of the body's natural 'foot-pump'. They studied the venous return of the healthy foot of Dr. Gardner using a non-irritant, painless, contrast media which was injected into a vein on the dorsum of the foot with the volunteer standing on his other foot.

In the erect posture and non weight-bearing the osmolar contrast media, that had been injected into the superficial vein of the dorsum of the foot, flowed distally (outwards) via a channel between the second and third metatarsal bases and pooled in two deep medial plantar veins and in the superficial tributaries; the most posterior of these was large and plexiform. Ankle or toe movements had no effect upon these veins but, on weight-bearing, the emptying was described as dramatic.

During normal ambulation, this filling and emptying action is repeated many times, in fact with every stride we take. Hence the medical truth in the old saying that 'walking is good for you'. This view is also held in China where the value of walking regularly is recognised generally. Or is it because they cannot get buses up their mountains?!

To return to our foot-pump: we now know that it not only empties up through the deep veins but also can empty through the long and short saphenous veins but not into other subcutaneous venous plexuses. Also, when walking, the action of the pump is synchronised with two further pumps situated in the calf muscles. There are other venous pumps and these are illustrated by Figure 13. Each is capable of dislocating a column of blood all the way up to the heart against the downward force of gravity.

There is one interesting difference between the foot-pump and the calf pumps. Whereas the foot-pump is not affected by ankle or toe movement, these movements do affect the calf pumps. The deep intramuscular veins in the lower calf empty upwards on dorsiflexion of the ankle. On plantarflexion, these veins fill from the superficial long saphenous vein via those that perforate the fascia of the calf.

Consequently, the pump and weight-bearing are important factors in the venous return of the lower limbs. Conversely, if weight-bearing is denied - either by illness or injury forcing the person to remain supine - venous return is impaired. This realisation led to the development of a devise that simulated the beneficial action of ambulation - a pneumatic pump.

Clinically, the pneumatic pump that was capable of being incorporated into an immobilising cast or slipper, proved very effective in reducing swelling after injury. An unexpected bonus was that it also reduced pain. Although, if it reduced swelling, one would expect some pain-reduction because of reduced pressure on the sensory nerves.

The pneumatic pump was used with great benefit in cases of ankle fracture, fractured tibia and in the avoidance of thromboses. I understand it is used now pre-operatively and throughout surgery and beyond in some of our major hospitals in the UK.

In another study of the venous return from the foot - by Lea Thomas in 1982 - it was stated that: " ... in contrast to the situation in the rest of the leg, veins of the foot have no haemodynamic importance". (From Phlebology 1985, D. Negus & G. Jantet© 1986, John Libbey & Co. Ltd.).

It was the use of videophlebography and the advent of a safe and painless osmolar contrast media that permitted the study and the proper understanding of the haemodynamics.

The previously held view, I believe, gives us a clue to why the established medical profession has found it so difficult to accept any efficacious outcome from the therapy of reflexology. Equally, the findings of Drs. Gardner and Fox gives an indication of how a good reflexology treatment assists blood circulation - each pressure/release action of finger or thumb around the foot and ankle areas act as miniature vascular 'pumps' of brief duration.

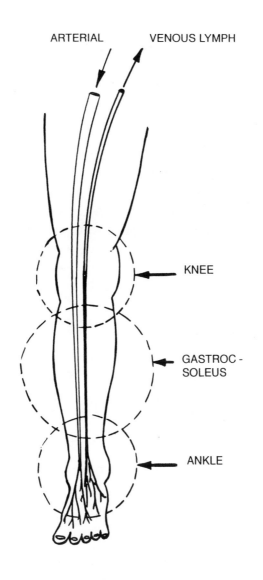

FIG 13: VASCULAR 'PUMPS' ~ LOWER LIMB

CHAPTER IV

CONDITIONS OF THE FEET, NAILS AND LOWER LIMBS

Conditions of the Feet

Deviated Big Toe (Hallux Valgus)   The big toe turns inwards, towards the centre-line of the foot - it is adducted - and remains in that position because bone, ligaments, muscle and adjacent tissue adjust to the abnormal position over a period of time.

Bunion is, simply, a bursa-sack of fluid - over a hallux valgus. The fluid often solidifies into a jelly-like substance before hardening further, with consequent increase in pain locally (Figure 14).

Mallet or Claw Toes   The distal phalanx of the toe remains in a plantarflexed position - in other words, the distal portion of the toe remains turned downwards, rather like a mallet or claw (Figure 15).

Hammer Toes   are where the proximal phalanx is bent upwards and the distal bone is bent downwards - forming a crude approximation to the shape of a hammer-head (Figure 15).

Webbed Toes   are those which are joined together, either from birth (hereditary) or as a result of an injury or serious burn. Usually, it is the second and third toes that are joined, either at their root or along their complete length. Obviously, shoes that are too narrow are totally inappropriate for this condition (Figure 15).

Flat Foot (Pes Plano Valgus) is a condition in which the medial longitudinal arch is lowered or flat, accompanied by eversion of the foot (Figure 16). It may be compounded by the collapse of the anterior transverse arch.

Factors that can lead to flat feet are:

- the ligaments and muscles become weak (overweight is one cause);
- the ligaments and muscles have become tired (overweight, prolonged standing contribute to this);
- body weight exceeds muscular and skeletal development (toddlers and teenagers are prone to this condition);
- spasm of the peroneal muscles (those in the calf), causing 'spastic flat foot'.

Footwear re flat feet:

The upper should not be too tight or too inflexible.

Free movement of the toes - particularly the big toe - is vital. Fitting is as important as shoe size - there is a natural temptation to go up a size for extra comfort, thereby having shoes that are too large to fit properly.

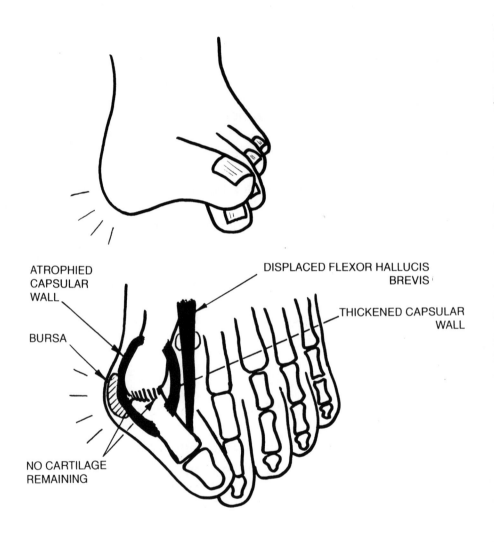

ATROPHIED CAPSULAR WALL

DISPLACED FLEXOR HALLUCIS BREVIS

THICKENED CAPSULAR WALL

BURSA

NO CARTILAGE REMAINING

FIG 14: A BUNION
(BURSA OVER A HALLUX VALGUS)

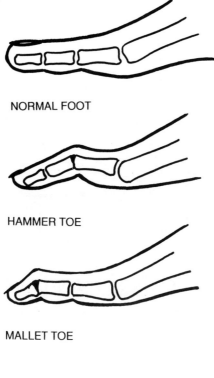

NORMAL FOOT

HAMMER TOE

MALLET TOE

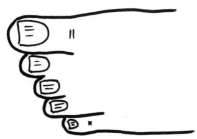

WEBBED TOES

FIG 15: CONDITIONS OF THE FEET

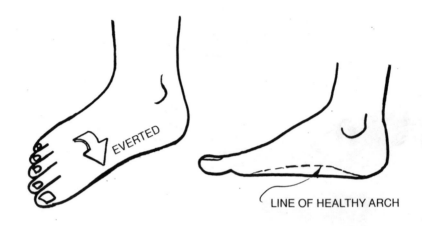

FIG 16: FLAT FOOT (PES PLANUS VALGUS)

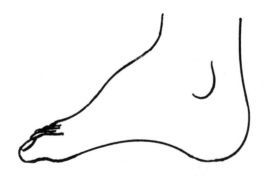

**FIG 17: ABNORMALLY HIGH ARCH
(PES CAVUS VALGUS)**

The sole should be a little larger than the foot when spread under full standing weight.

The inner border should be straight and the heel sole horizontal.

The shoe should be a snug fit with the instep of the foot - see 'Star Quality Fitting', Figure 23 and also 'Fit to Wear and Fit for Comfort', Figure 24.

The patient/customer should be advised against socks or stockings that cramp the natural spread of the toes - thus nullifying the healthy advantages of a well-fitted shoe.

Abnormally High Instep & Arch, i.e. Pes Cavus Valgus of the foot is an unusually high longitudinal arch (Figure 17). When walking, all the weight is via the balls of the feet - metatarsal heads - causing considerable discomfort, particularly over the first and fifth metatarsal heads; all the toes are clawed. Often the condition is associated with other medical problems, e.g. spina bifida and polio.

It is difficult to get shoes deep enough to accommodate this type of foot. But every effort should be made to obtain shoes that are sufficiently deep and wide to allow pressure-relieving padding and appliances to be fitted to alleviate much of the discomfort.

Heel Pain

Calcaneal Spur (Figure 18)   Normally this causes discomfort only when standing or walking - the pain can vary from a dull ache to extremely intense: it is more common amongst people of middle years or older.

Bursitis is a sac of fluid below the skin which has become inflamed. Common sites are at a bunion - strictly speaking, a bunion is bursitis of a hallux valgus - and at the back of the heel, when it is called **Cancaneal Bursitis** (Figure 18).

Posterior Cancaneal Bursitis (Figure 18) is inflammation of the bursa located between the Archilles tendon and the skin. Usually, this condition is caused by friction from ill-fitting shoes - particularly amongst women who wear high heeled shoes!

Hyperhidrosis (sweaty feet) and Bromidrosis (smelly feet)

One or both of these foot conditions can be caused by hormonal changes and the condition, therefore, is more common amongst adolescents and may occur in some women at menopause.

Generally, sufferers need good foot hygiene - regular washing in tepid water, thorough drying - particularly between all toes - plus dusting the feet daily with a proprietry antifungal powder, e.g. 'Mycil', 'Dactarin', 'Phytocil' ... Care is needed to dust the feet as distinct from smothering the feet - which simply blocks the pores of the skin with powder.

Footwear - cotton socks in summer, changed at least once every day; woollen socks in colder weather and shoes of leather - allowing the feet to 'breathe' - in preference to synthetic materials.

Callouses are areas of hard skin that build up in response to friction and/or pressure - they are nature's responsive protection.

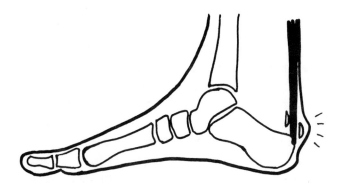

CALCANEAL BURSITIS (POSTERIOR)

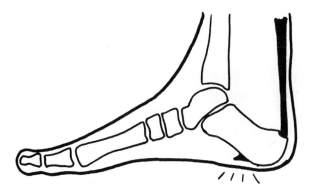

CALCANEAL SPUR

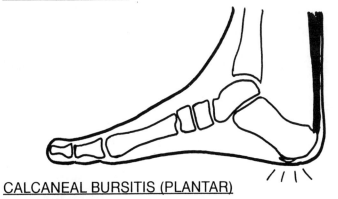

CALCANEAL BURSITIS (PLANTAR)

FIG 18: HEEL PAIN

<u>Corns</u> are a local, painful, development of a callous. Often they form over a bony prominence and result from pressure and slight friction, as caused by shoes that 'pinch' the feet. The callous builds up in one tiny spot and pressure prevents its spread, so the layers build one upon another, driving into the foot because the footwear resists the upward and outward growth. They feel as if there is a splinter in the foot and indeed the core of a dry corn (Heloma Durum) is very similar in texture to a small piece of timber.

A qualified Chiropodist can remove (enucleate) corns and remove the pain but not necessarily the cause! That depends upon our willingness to buy shoes that are well designed for healthy living and that are fitted properly, together with well fitting socks, stockings or tights.

<u>Soft interdigital corns (Heloma Molle)</u>   A soft corn is a macerated overgrowth of the outer layer of skin (epidermis) that occurs usually between the toes - often between toes four and five and on the side of one of them.

They have a white, rubbery appearance - the localised mass distinguishing it from 'athletes foot' (tinea pedis).

An initial indication of a soft corn is when the patient complains of a burning sensation between the toes. Later it produces the sensation of a small stone or a few grains of sand or grit; it is a prickly/smarting pain and it has been known for the skin to break to leave a pin hole.

<u>Verrucae</u>   are warts, usually on the plantar (underneath) surface of the feet; they are more common amongst children and young people and amongst adults who play a lot of sport - particularly swimming, squash, badminton, etc. all of which involve frequent use of shared changing facilities.

Verrucae are believed to be caused by a virus infection which invades the outer layers of skin (the dermis and epidermis). They vary in size from a pin head to the size of a pencil-top and can, if neglected, spread to the size of a 5p piece. They can be extremely painful and they are distinguished by characteristic little reddish/brown dots; they can be soft, spongy, moist, dry, raised or flat.

Treatment: sometimes they will disappear spontaneously but usually they require some encouragement in the form of treatment by a qualified chiropodist or by a General Practitioner familiar with the various treatments and with the peculiarities of the condition. They are extremely infectious and must, therefore, be kept dry and isolated during treatment and until they have disappeared completely and are replaced by healthy tissue.

Dropped Metatarsal Arch

One of the most common conditions presented to a therapist is the dropped metatarsal arch or 'splay foot' - Figure 20. The patient complains of pain under the metatarsal heads when they are weight-bearing.

Golfers are prone to the condition. The right-handed player will have the problem usually affecting the left foot. The golf swing - when executed properly - transfers the weight from the back foot to the left foot. Repetition of this movement causes a problem in those predisposed to it, i.e. overweight, lacking regular alternative exercise or those with an inherent weakness.

The pain can be quite severe - as if walking on pebbles and/or of a burning nature. It can cause considerable worry about the ability to continue to play sport or the longer term threat to the quality of life. Sometimes a patient will tell us that they have to sleep with their feet outside the bed covers - to ease the burning sensation.

Women who wear high-heeled shoes habitually are more prone to the condition than men. High heeled shoes throw a greater proportion of the body's weight on to the metatarsal heads - Figure 19 below.

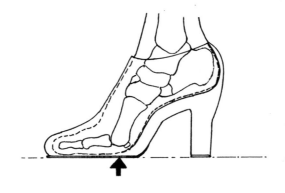

FIG 19: MOST OF BODY-WEIGHT ON METATARSAL HEADS

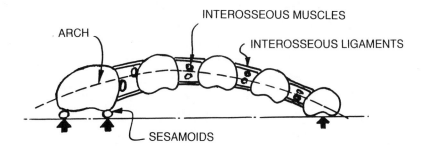

STATIC FOOT ~ METATARSAL ARCH

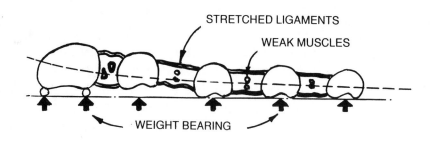

FIG 20: STATIC FOOT ~ COLLAPSED ARCH OR 'SPLAY FOOT'

In a healthy foot the configuration is that the anterior heads of the metatarsal bones form the metatarsal arch.

When standing, the first and fifth metatarsal heads rest on the floor or ground; whilst the second, third and fourth metatarsal heads are raised to form a shallow arch (Figure 20). The majority of the bodyweight is borne by the first metatarsal - the largest and strongest of these bones. Much of the rest of the bodyweight is supported by the fifth metatarsal - the second largest of the metatarsals. The rest of the bodyweight is spread between the other three bones. With a fallen arch these same three bones are forced to withstand an increased proportion of the total weight.

In addition to the continual wearing of high-heeled shoes, other factors that contribute are slack supporting muscles - often due to the inactivity of a long illness or to an incapacitating injury; jobs involving long hours standing - policemen, teachers, bank cashiers, shop assistants .....

The condition can be recognised quite easily. The inner metatarsal heads bulge instead of being raised in an arch. They may be red and warm - indicating inflammation - pressure applied with the thumb to the plantar aspect of the fourth metatarsal produces a sharp, stabbing, pain. Because the arch has dropped, the four smaller toes will be plantar flexed slightly and may have callouses or even corns over the proximal phalangeal joints. Also, there are calluses under the first and fifth metatarso - phalangeal joints. In chronic cases, there may be arthritis affecting the metatarso-phalangeal joints.

Treatment

The primary aim is to relieve the pain, followed by correction and re-toning of the associated muscles, to sustain the improved condition and to reduce the chances of a recurrence.

In the case of corns and callouses that may be present, refer the patient to a qualified chiropodist who will enucleate the corns and pare down the callouses.

It is now necessary to apply padding and strapping to prevent pressure on the parts treated by the chiropodist - who may correct the dropped arch condition in addition to the surgical work. Whoever undertakes the task, the procedure is as follows: a metatarsal pad is cut from adhesive felt of approximately 7 millimetres thick to the shape (shown in Figure 21, a to d). The width of the anterior part of the pad must be sufficient to support the second, third and fourth metatarsals. The edges should be chamfered, using scissors, to produce a smooth and even edge to the pad. Notice also that the pad is sloped posteriorly (Figure 21b). Strip away the adhesive covering and apply the pad to the plantar surface of the foot so that the anterior edge is positioned just posterior (below, as you look at the plantar or underside of the foot) to the metatarsal heads. The pad is held in place with three strips of adhesive tape, as shown. The ends of the strapping are well rounded, to prevent them coming unstuck. The pad is kept in place for a week, when the patient is seen again - to check progress - and the padding procedure is repeated.

The effect of the pad is to raise metatarsal heads two, three and four. The action of walking acts also as a further self-correction: the patient's arch is lifted gently and pulled into its correct position with every step that the patient takes.

The relief from these initial measures can be quite dramatic. Once the patient gets used to the feel of the padding, they will be able to walk without pain and be oblivious to the pads.

At the return visit, the second treatment, the foot is massaged thoroughly to continue or enhance the reduction in swelling and to restore mobility to the forefoot, reduce adhesions and to nourish the tissue-cells. The reflexologist's diaphragm relaxing move is also a very beneficial form of forefoot loosening. This, combined with deep friction and effleurage massage and vigorous shaking of the metatarsals, will keep the foot supple.

In my experience, padding for four weeks, followed by faradic foot baths for a further four weeks, usually is sufficient to correct a collapsed metatarsal arch. Once again, the gratitude of the patient for the relief of pain and the restoration of healthy mobility is sufficient to make the therapist also feel better!

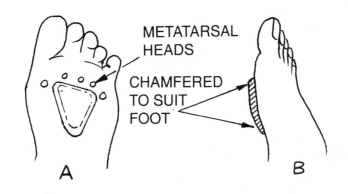

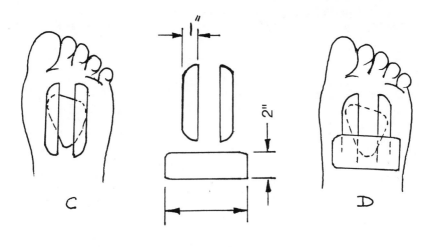

TO SUIT FOOT-WIDTH

FIG 21: METATARSAL PADDING TO RELIEVE DROPPED ARCH

48

Nail Conditions

Condition	Aetiology	Treatment
Onychauxis (abnormal thickening) from root to margin. Often accompanied by dark yellow/brown discolouration	Matrix damaged by: - trauma, - neglect of trimming, - fungi, - systemic disturbance	Reduce thickness of nail with burrs; check footwear; regular treatment necessary
Onychocryptosis (in growing) often with swelling, inflammation and/or sepsis	Hyperdrosis; faulty nail-cutting; ill-fitting footwear	Remove wedge of nail; smooth cut edge with Black's file; apply suitable antiseptic; maybe cover with tubigauze
Onychogryphosis (Ram's Horn or Ostler's Toe) thickening of nail plus deformity in shape of ram's horn	As onychauxis, with trauma most common cause	Reduce nail with nippers and burrs - care needed to avoid haemorrhage from tissue caught up in nail
Onychophosis (calloused and/or sore sulci) sulci swollen, inflamed and may contain heloma	Lateral pressure from footwear and/or adjacent valgus; lack of smoothing after nail-cutting; harsh probing of sulci	Soften sulci (Hydro. Perox. 10 vol. solution); remove callous; enucleate any heloma; smooth lateral edges of nail; apply antiseptic
Paronychia ('Whitlow' - inflamed tissue surrounding nail plate)	Any trauma that facilitates entry of foreign body or bacteria. Unskilled nail-care	Acute: reduce inflammation with hot (115°C max.) saline bath; apply antiseptic and protective dressing and rest the foot until symptoms subside. Chronic: patient to repeat bathing, as above, every 4 hrs until all pus has drained and report back for check, antiseptic and protective dressing. If nil response to treatment in 48 hrs, **refer to GP**
Onychia (inflamed matrix) often occurs with above condition and vice versa	As above	As above
Onycholysis (separation of nail plate from matrix) elderly most susceptible	Skin conditions, e.g. psoriasis, eczema: systemic condition/s or trauma	Irrigate; cut nail away; seal with Acritensil or New Skin, to prevent infection. If systemic condition suspected, **refer to GP**

Condition	Aetiology	Treatment
Onychomadesis (complete nail-plate loss)	Severe trauma or constitutional disorder	Clean area thoroughly; seal to prevent infection; consider fitting false nail: if cause not trauma, refer to GP re possible constitutional problem
Onychatrophia (retarded nail-growth) can lead to Onychomadesis	Debilitating illness; skin disease; old age; severe constitutional disorder	Refer to GP re probable constitutional disorder or if skin disease evident
Onychomycosis (fungal infection) nail becomes brittle, thickened, opaque and brownish yellow in colour: nail not as thickened as with Onychauxis	Difficult to be precise, predisposition would be poor foot hygiene, adjacent skin infection or cross infection from public footbaths, etc.	Regular use of fungicide, e.g. Phytex Paint. Treatment can take many months re: slow nail replacement rate. If adjacent skin infection, **refer to GP**
Onychorrhexis (splitting and/or brittle nails) often with distinct longitudinal ridging	Can occur with ageing or result from constitutional disorder, e.g. anaemia, rheumatism. Can be due to mal-absorption of vitamins and/or calcium, zinc or magnesium deficiency	Care when trimming nails and use of suitable sealant post op. to minimise further splitting
Koilonychia (spooned shaped nail/s)	Often **Diabetes Mellitus**. Also, can be due to debilitating deficiency such as anaemia	Re: diabetes mellitus, check shape of finger nails. Trim tow-nails **with great care**. If patient not know diabetic, refer to GP for tests. Also refer if debilitating deficiency suspected.
Beau's Lines (transverse ridges across width of nail-plate)	Some past constitutional disorder causing temporary arrest of nail growth	Resolves itself - lines appear first at root and advance with normal growth of nail-plate
Hippocratic Nails (club nails) can extend over apex of toe/s	Frequently associated with chronic cardiac or pulmonary condition	Care needed to avoid pain when nail is trimmed back: otherwise observe the note
White Spots on Nails	Can be from previous localised trauma or can be one sign of deficiency in zinc or vitamin A	Observe and note only

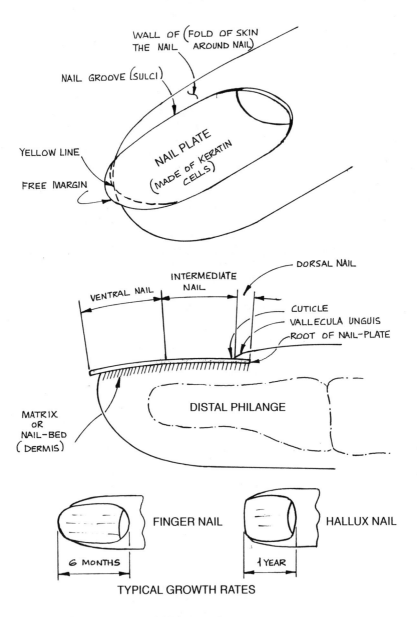

WALL OF (FOLD OF SKIN
THE NAIL AROUND NAIL)

NAIL GROOVE (SULCI)

YELLOW LINE

FREE MARGIN

NAIL PLATE
(MADE OF KERATIN CELLS)

VENTRAL NAIL

INTERMEDIATE NAIL

DORSAL NAIL

CUTICLE
VALLECULA UNGUIS
ROOT OF NAIL-PLATE

DISTAL PHILANGE

MATRIX
OR
NAIL-BED
(DERMIS)

FINGER NAIL

HALLUX NAIL

6 MONTHS

1 YEAR

TYPICAL GROWTH RATES

FIG 22: ANATOMY OF THE NAIL

Leg Ulcers

Introduction

This topic has been included, despite it being above the foot, because it causes so much pain and distress to the sufferers. Women, in particular, are embarrassed often by having to wear bandages that they regard as unsightly and uncomfortable.

A leg ulcer is the result of the advanced stage of failure of the peripheral circulation.

Historically, they were called 'living wounds' because they lasted only as long as the patient!

Many ulcerated conditions last for many years and occupy the attention and care of General Practitioners and District Nurses (if that is still their title!). This costs society not only the loss of working days and the cost of medical and nursing care, but also a considerable cost in dressing materials alone.

It has been estimated by some specialists that 80% of leg ulcers are due to a varicose condition. The remaining 20% is made up of diabetes, cardiovascular conditions, kidney disease, venereal disease and extremely poor nutrition.

Causes

Most ulcers result from a chronic existing circulatory condition, such as deep vein thrombosis (DVT), arterial sclerosis, occlusion or varicosity. Consequently, ulcers arising from any of these pre-disposing conditions have a chronic origin (excluding those arising from traumatic or post-operative causes).

A summary of some of the causes is as follows:

Internal - DVT - often post-natal or post-surgery.
In each situation the body is static, supine
and the whole of the lymphatic and
circulatory system is allowed to become
sluggish
- Arterial sclerosis
- Chronic asthma
- Allergies to some antibiotics
- Extreme obesity
- Constipation
- Bad posture
Injury - Pelvic damage
- Replacement hip/s
- Burns
- Insect bites

A thrombus can be removed surgically. It is quite hard and
can be the size of a pea. Once removed, often from above
the site of an ulcer, healing accelerates considerably.

Development of an Ulcer

Ulcers are caused by varicose blocking of valves - they
become clogged by stagnant platelets - and this leads to the
platelets being formed outside the lymphatic venous system
and under the skin. This causes minor infection and irritation,
leading to eczema which, in turn, can develop into the forma-
tion of an ulcer.

Arterial ulcers ascend legs, varicose ulcers descend legs.
The signs and symptoms of arterial ulcers are that they are
usually superficial, always dry, have no odour and they have
a bluish rim to them. However, they can be extremely painful

and even bed covers resting on the affected area can be painful to the patient. In contrast, varicose ulcers can be extremely deep, even to the depth of the bone.

Varicose Ulcer - Stages of Development

1. Impaired or sluggish venous return. Venous dilation; breakdown of valves causing reflux of venous blood - resulting in dilated, incompetent veins of lower limb.
2. Sediment of fragments of platelets and of erythrocytes escape into the subcutaneous tissue - causing the break-down of the epidermis and local discolouration, skin-irritation, leading to:
3. Eczema (wet and dry forms) and then:
4. Varicose ulcer

Arterial Ulcer - Development

Usually starts at the distal part of the affected limb - at the heel or toes. The pre-disposing causes are either

- arterial sclerosis (hardening of the artery), or
- an occlusion - usually a thrombus in the sub-popliteal artery.

The latter cause is frequent amongst chronic and heavy smokers.

Observation

Is there any oedema?
Are there bags under the eyes?
Is the patient obese?
Is there any malfunction of movement?
Do the feet turn inwards or outwards?
 (N.B. venous ulcers - the patient turns the foot inwards -
 adducts; arterial ulcers - the patient limps)
Is there evidence of arthritis?
Does the patient's posture appear inadequate in any way?
Note appearance and condition of skin and hair.
Note appearance and location of the ulcer, its size, any
 discharge?

Examination

Is the patient diabetic?
Check the patient's blood pressure.
Test the urine - Clinistix can be purchased from chemists and
 the test can reveal a number of characteristics, including
 alkaline level (pH), glucose, blood, protein, ketones, etc.
Check current medication.
Check length of time on medication - effect can be
 cumulative.
Check the patient's diet.
Check the patient's bowel habits, chronic constipation clogs
 the descending colon and, consequently, causes adverse
 venal pressure.
Examine the limb for thrombosed nodules.

Treatment

Must be by a Registered Medical Physician and would include:

- Exercise, within the limitations of the patient, their current general health and their age.
- Elevation of the limb and the application of bandaging, as follows: Apply Tubigauze, or its equivalent, from toe to knee. Roll Tubigauze back down leg, to expose ulceration. Apply cream or ointment as applicable - if there is a discharge, use cream - ointment is suitable for dry lesions. Using sterile forceps, apply three double layers of Vaseline gauze or iodine. Apply Melolin dressing. Finally, apply elasticated, flesh-coloured, Tubigrip bandage or an equivalent flesh coloured covering.

It must be born in mind that the treatment of ulcers remains individual; what suits one patient can prove to be unsuitable for another - even within the same family. A good firm bandaging technique, however, forms an important part of effective treatment.

The foregoing is intended as a general guide and is shared information. **It is not intended to replace the knowledge and judgement of registered medical physicians who should be the persons consulted in all ulcerative conditions.**

Nutrition

A 'good' diet helps - as with all aspects of good health. Good, in the context of either reducing the chance of an ulcer or in assisting recovery, would be a diet rich in fruit, fibre, vegetables, minerals and vitamins, with adequate daily consumption of spring water or filtered water. The other side of the same diet-coin would be less strong coffee and tea (try herb teas instead), less animal fats, sweets, cakes and puddings. If obese, have less of everything! Smoking should be avoided.

Apparently, very few vegetarians get leg ulcers.

Again, it cannot be emphasised too strongly that the nutritional aspects must be tailored to suit the individual constitution of each patient and the outcomes must be monitored by those qualified to do so.

Mr. Nigel Vukovich, SRN, RMN, NDN, DO, noticed a difference in the incidence of ulcers within the UK population. There is a difference between the rural and the city population. Presumably, city dwellers tend to walk less often and for shorter distances than their country cousins. Very few manual works, for example, have leg ulcers.

I hereby gratefully acknowledge the help and advice given to me by Mr. Vukovich. Much of this section on leg ulcers is based largely upon his great experience and generosity. I trust that the pleasure gained by sharing experience for the benefit of others is mutual.

CHAPTER V

SPORTS INJURIES TO THE FOOT & ANKLE

Fifteen or twenty years ago sports injuries were associated with contact sports and spare-time outdoor pursuits or indoor gymnastics. Today, many more people are attending fitness centres that are an integral part of community leisure centres or that are attached to large hotels. Consequently, the opportunities to injure ourselves are greater now in an age where physical fitness is more fashionable than in previous decades. Paradoxically, there are more sedentary occupations than previously, so the need to make a special effort to exercise has replaced our more energetic past. This not only applies to adults! I shudder to think what problems the children of today are storing by a general lack of physical exercise in their everyday lives. They are taken to school and collected from school by car. Many sports fields attached to or owned by schools have been sold to developers and physical education no longer seems to be an accepted integral and frequent part of a school's weekly timetable.

We are moving towards the physical contrast between static situations interspersed with often sudden or violent activity. Failure to allow time to warm up will increase the incidence of muscle injuries. In addition, those who become addicted to fitness tighten muscles to such an extent that there is little residual elasticity and, consequently, pulled muscles and/or torn tendons become an increased risk. Once again, we must balance how much we exercise and what type of exercise and how frequently we exercise: if we walk or cycle instead of driving or riding we do ourselves a health favour.

Medical Records

Therapists, whether 'orthodox' or complementary, must note what sports are played by a patient and how frequently. Also note other activities and pastimes (that they will admit!). Even the game of chess can influence musculoskeletal structure: the way a patient sits habitually affects posture and structure and, therefore, the condition and flexibility of the lower limbs and feet. For example, people who sit with feet crossed (not just legs crossed) often complain of a 'dead spot' on their instep.

Observe the patient's every movement - do they rise from a chair like some space rocket or do they first lean forward slightly and, keeping their spine straight, come up and out of the chair gracefully, using their leg muscles in a co-ordinated, smooth, movement?

Bruising

With today's ultra light weight boots worn by soccer and rugby players, a common injury is bruising under a toe nail - usually under the nail of the big toe (hallux).

A bruise is a localised area of damaged blood vessels that leak blood into surrounding tissue: gradually this blood is carried away by our body, whilst the bruise undergoes its familiar sequence of colour changes.

A bruise under a nail is particularly painful because the leaked blood has nowhere to go so the pressure builds under the nail. If the throbbing pain is severe and difficult to tolerate, action is necessary before the blood under the nail has time to congeal.

There are two methods used by chiropodists. One is the gentle use of a red hot fine needle to burn through the nail carefully and thus puncture the trapped pocket of blood, releasing the pressure and providing instant reduction of pain. The second method is exactly the same principle, but instead of a red hot needle, a high speed, fine, burr is used to drill a release hole very gently through the nail. In either case, the released blood will shoot into the air like a fountain, under the force of pressure under the nail. The instant pain-relief puts a smile back on the face of the sufferer.

Bruising elsewhere on the foot or ankle, due to an over zealous opponent, or the advancing years slowing avoiding action, can be treated by hot and cold compresses applied alternately for about ten minutes, two or three times a day. This will encourage the blood-flow locally, reduce swelling and reduce pain. **If the bruising is such that the foot or ankle has lost mobility - consult your doctor immediately. Equally, if the 'bruise' looks like a large blood blister, consult your doctor because it is likely to be a swelling of congested blood, called a haematoma which requires medical care to avoid a possible thrombosis (blood clot).**

Digital Sprain

Stubbing the toe or persistent hyperflexion (bending) as in golf, squash and jogging can lead to digital sprain. Running on hard, unyielding surfaces or an uneven terrain puts additional strain on the feet. Remember that when running, our contact foot momentarily has to withstand over three times our body-weight and, at toe-off, the toes have to take that total weight.

Signs and Symptoms: pain and swelling at the metatarsopha-langeal joint or interphalangeal joint.   Occasionally, erectus spasm of the toe in hyperdorsiflexion, i.e. when the toe is bent to an extreme position it goes into spasm and sticks up and is very painful, can be released by applying warmth/heat to toe.

Secondary Effects: capsulitis (inflammation of the joint cap-sule) or stress fracture may follow digital sprain or coincide with it.

- Pain at rest - digital sprain indicated.
- Pain with movement - digital sprain, with capsulitis indi-cated.

Treatment: the standard 'RICE' procedure of:

- Rest.
- Ice - if seen within 24hrs of the trauma.
- Compression (bandaging).
- Elevation (raise legs above level of trunk).

If no movement after 72hrs, **refer** to GP for possible X-ray.

If seen more than 24hrs after trauma, use hot and cold compresses alternately - to diffuse tissue-congestion, oede-matus fluid around site and to encourage circulation and lymphatic drainage.

N.B.   If toe has no mobility, with severe pain, **refer immedi-ately** to doctor or nearest Accident & Emergency Unit.

Tendonitis (inflamed tendon/s)

This condition may be due to the causes of digital sprain or to ill-fitting footwear. Check by taking the foot or toe through the full range of normal movement, whilst simultaneously palpating the tendon. **Do not tell the patient what you are doing,** instead, **ask how it feels** (not does it hurt?!). It is equally important - as with reflexology - to watch the patient's facial expression whilst moving the affected part!

Treatment:

- Reduce inflammation.
- Ice and rest as much as circumstances allow, total rest is preferable.

If in doubt refer to a doctor or to a qualified chiropodist.

Metatarsalgia

This is a general term that embraces the following conditions:

Sesamoiditis - trauma of the sesamoids (the bones that act as 'ball-bearings' easing the movement of a joint - particularly at the first metatarsophalangeal joint). Ballet dancers are prone to this condition as are over enthusiastic aerobic devotees: it is a very painful condition.

Bursitis - an inflamed and swollen bursa (sack of synovial fluid at back and underneath calcaneum bone).

Neuroma - a nodular, benign growth, usually in the inter-metatarsal region.

Capsulitis - inflammation of the capsule between a joint and its articulate cartilage.

Stress fracture - often at the third metatarsal bone and caused by 'normal' but repetitive and persistent stress - see also

Treatment section. This condition occurs, primarily, with runners and young footballers (Figure 23).

Dislocation - total misalignment of joint surfaces: toes most often effected. These are re-aligned by pulling the toe (to gap the joint) and appropriate pressure locally to 'spring' the joint back into line. Pain is severe but brief, followed by great probability of bad language from the patient and then aching pain until swelling and any local inflammation subsides.

Subluxation (a term used also for certain types of spinal misalignment) - partial dislocation. Occasionally, a patient can self-correct: immediate remedial action is desirable before joint swells and/or becomes inflamed.

Treatment

Sesamoiditis - fitting of a palliative orthotic to prevent further trauma to the area: this must be done by a qualified chiropodist, physiotherapist or doctor.

Bursitis - cold therapy; application of anti inflammatory, for example 1% hydrocortisone - therefore, refer patient to their General Practitioner.

Neuroma - palpate to diagnose; it has a 'rolled up sock' feel. Compare other interdigital areas; prescribe rest and refer to patient's General Practitioner for probable invasive surgery to remove the nodule (as with **Morton's neuroma**).

Capsulitis - check dorsiflexion of toe and palpate over the joint.

Stress Fracture

Usually occurs at second or third metatarsal bone (see Figure 23). Wear and tear exceeds bone replacement process **or osteoclastic** (the cells which dissolves or removes unwanted bone cells) activity exceeds the **osteoblastic** (bone forming cells) activity. When the osteoclastic process is greater than the osteoblastic process, a weakness develops and eventually the bone cracks under stress. Sometimes, it may not be noticeable until about three weeks after the incident. Inadequate diet and/or inadequate hormone secretion can contribute to the increased chance of suffering this type of injury.

Clinical signs/symptoms: pain/redness over dorsal (upper) aspect of the foot area, aggravated by movement and there is diffuse swelling.

Treatment: rest for approximately three weeks - to decrease flexion (bending) at metatarso/phalangeal joints - wooden clogs are ideal footwear to assist this inactivity and to minimise damage to the metatarsals and phalanges. After three weeks, introduce shoe with metatarsal pad, for further three weeks. After six weeks, condition should have healed, when a functional orthotic can be applied.

Dislocation & Subluxation

Before any manipulation, determine age of injury (to avoid tearing tendons, ligaments, etc.). **Must** massage joint before manipulation and again afterwards - to adjust muscle to 'new' normal alignment: ensure patient rests for minimum of ten minutes after treatment (re: pain and shock). When swelling and pain have subsided, check range of movement is back to normal, compare with corresponding, undamaged, normal movement.

With an **old** injury, two massage treatments, before repositioning is attempted. Care is needed to avoid re-injuring after manipulation.

Heel-Spur Syndrome

Caused by nerve entrapment, exostosis (an overgrowth of bone tissue forming a tumour), arthritis, neuritis, inadequate footwear, calcaneal stress fracture; an insufficient fatty pad (in elderly, AIDS sufferers and cancer patients).

Check by palpating plantar area with **both** thumb pads - gentle push simulates walking pressure/action and hard push simulates jogging, etc.

Treatment - application of orthotic sponge heel pad - with hole; correction of gait; modification of footwear; sponge heel pad without cut-out (re. insufficient fatty pad); cold or heat application, to stimulate local circulation.

Soft Tissue Injury of Posterior Foot

Calcaneodynia (heel pain)

Anorexic people may suffer this condition because tissue shrinkage intensifies the pain. Similarly, it can affect the elderly, cancer patients and AIDS sufferers and can lead to ulceration.

Treatment - palliative padding, plus refer to general practitioner for systemic evaluation.

Plantar Fat Pad Syndrome

Occurs at site proximal to where heel spur might be and anterior to that spot (just posterior to mid-tarsal region, or

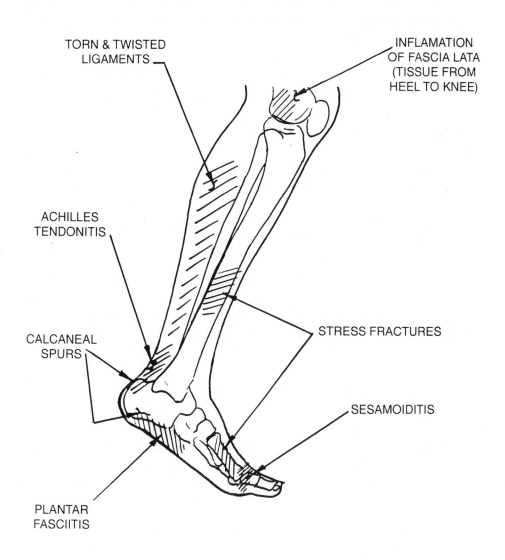

TORN & TWISTED
LIGAMENTS

INFLAMATION
OF FASCIA LATA
(TISSUE FROM
HEEL TO KNEE)

ACHILLES
TENDONITIS

STRESS FRACTURES

CALCANEAL
SPURS

SESAMOIDITIS

PLANTAR
FASCIITIS

FIG 23: SPORTS RELATED INJURIES-
THEIR LOCATION & TYPE

arch of foot). Inflammation of pad; abnormal pronation (over an inner border, i.e. heel-strike-to-inner, instead of heel-strike-to-outer movement of foot).

Diagnosis - cream on hand and rub over area; on contact, patient experiences pain, i.e. you palpate the plantar mass.

Plantar Fasciitis

Inflammation of the fascia due to chronic, repetitive stress; usually as a result of an acute injury, leading to rupture. In chronic cases, the ruptures attract scar tissue and these 'lumps' can be detected when you palpate the area. Found, usually, in plantar mid-foot area.

Treatment - apply crepe bandage in a 'figure of 8' wrapped around mid-foot to ankle - to 'lock' the mid tarsal area and to stop dorsiflexion. Can also wrap around hallux and back around ankle in 'figure of 8' configuration - to immobilise hallux, in addition to mid-tarsal area.

Inflamed Retro-Calcanean Exostosis

A large, red, lump on the back of the heel caused by short shoes or boots. Also, can be due to poorly fitted running shoes. Can pad over area, to remove irritation. If severe, refer to general practitioner for probable bone reduction by invasive surgery.

Examination/Assessment   'SOAP' philosophy, i.e.

Subjective - what the patient tells us
Objective - what we observe about the patient and condition
Assessment - what we judge/diagnose
Plan - programme of treatment/prognosis

Check

1. Inspect, **don't touch** initially.
2. Palpation.
3. Temperature - pyrexia (fever temperature).
4. Oedema.
5. Question **nature/type** of pain (get from patient, **don't lead**) e.g. does it pulsate (with heart-beat)? Is it sharp, dull, stabbing, intermittent, continuous or shooting (due to blood vessel restriction) ...?
6. **Range** of movement, compare to normal ...
7. Muscle power - 'APR' test, i.e. <u>A</u>ctive, <u>P</u>assive, <u>R</u>estrictive.
8. Joint stability.

<u>Plan - short term</u> - prevention of further damage, limitation of any haemorrhage, reduction of pain, reduction of oedema, prevention of immobility, stiffness in joints and tissue and maintenance of muscle-power.

<u>Plan - long term</u> - re-education of movement, restoration of function, increase muscle-power, prevention of return of oedema, prevention of re-occurrence of injury, increase mobility of joints and tissue and return to regular (normal) living.

Appliance Therapy

Paddings provide immobilisation of painful joints, deters friction, pressure and continued trauma, provides relief to weight-bearing areas and facilitates and accelerates the healing process of the traumatised area.

Dependant upon padding techniques, dorsiflexion and/or plantarflexion may be minimised deliberately and can cause acute change in foot bio-dynamics, leading to biomechanical disorder of the entire anatomy.   This refers to 'chairside' orthotics provided within a routine treatment-time.

Padding is quick, easy to make - possibly in one treatment session.   It has a useful life-span regarding the care of a patient and they can walk away with it in place and working immediately.

Contra Indications

- allergy to padding material,
- ability of patient to reach a detachable device, in such cases, fit to the **shoe,**
- may restrict circulation.

Procedure

- usually via toe or toes.

Selection

- thickness and grade of padding used, is determined by:

(a) effect required,
(b) volume and depth of footwear,
(c) limitation of normal movement of foot,
(d) type of footwear worn, e.g. useless with open-toed shoes or slip-ons,
(e) shoes where the wear is one-sided.

For checking depth of shoe, get patient to put their hand in shoe and wiggle to observe depth and spread of toes and to simulate foot movement. Note: width of adult hand usually equals width of foot (at metatarsal arch).

<u>Measurement</u> - (as normal part of procedure). Hold foot with hand across it and squeezing - to simulate shoe-pressure and make lateral measurement in this slightly restricted mode. This measurement must be entered on the patient's medical record, for future reference.

<u>Orthodigital Straightening of Toes</u>   The use of orthotics and re-alignment of toes is the work of a qualified chiropodist. Consequently, **complementary practitioners should refer their patient and not attempt to step outside their compe-tence or outside the parameters of the therapy in which they are trained and qualified.**

A few words on this topic are appropriate, however, as a small bridge of understanding.

The prime purpose is the correction and restoration of normal function, plus the protection of painful areas. Foot size has to be considered, together with the misalignment of the toes, before an application of orthodigital therapy. An assessment of the suitability of the patient's current shoes, socks or hosiery is assessed at the same time. It would be useless fitting corrective orthotics, if the cause, or contributo⁻ ause was the basic footwear. In this case that must be adᴗ essed and its outcome/progress assessed before moving on to the fitting of a specific orthotic device. Equally, suitable footwear can be valuable in assisting the corrective effect of an applied device.   It requires a comprehensive approach to restore normal function.

CHAPTER VI

DIABETES MELLITUS

It may seem strange that, in a book about feet, diabetes is featured. The reason is that those qualified in massage or indeed any of the touch therapies need to recognise the significance of diabetes. Qualified chiropodists are fully aware of the extra care needed when treating their diabetic patients.

Assuming our patient may not be aware that they are diabetic, the following signs would alert us to the possibility and to suggest that they should undergo a clinical assessment:

- slow healing of wounds or ulcers,
- calf-pain after walking only a short distance, e.g. 100/200 metres; known medically as intermittent claudication,
- tendency to limp because of the above discomfort,
- breath smells of pear drops (acidosis),
- numbness of extremities (peripheral neuropathy),
- cold feet, even in warm weather (impaired circulation),
- dark blue/black colour of toes (as with very cold feet),
- cataracts (retinopathy - damage caused by poor circulation),
- fatigue - gets tired more easily than we would expect,
- mood swings (due to varying blood-sugar levels),
- continuous thirst (polydipsia),
- weight-loss.

It must be stressed that we take these signs collectively and our suspicion would be aroused only when the majority of these signs are present. This is because, as in most aspects of health, signs can be indicative of other conditions. For example, calf-pain could be due to minor muscle strain; numbness of extremities applies also to Raynaud's Syndrome; cold feet (even in warm weather) is also a sign of hypothyroidism; dark blue/black toes can be frost-bite; cataracts might be familial and/or hereditary and fatigue and mood-swings (together with weight-gain) is associated with poor liver function and hypothyroidism or might be an early sign of a more serious condition. These possibilities serve to remind us that, if we suspect or are in any doubt, always **refer the patient to a registered medical physician.**

This is an appropriate time to take a closer look at the condition.

Certain cells in the alveoli of the pancreas - the beta cells of the Islets of Langerhans - produce insulin that enables the body tissues to oxidise glucose, that is absorbed from the bloodstream of the bowel, to form energy and to store glucose in muscle tissue in the form of glycogen. Insulin also regulates the metabolism of carbohydrates.

Therefore, the function of the pancreas is to produce just sufficient quantities of insulin to balance the needs of the body's tissues; to oxidise and store glucose and to keep the blood-sugar balanced to maintain good health.

If the pancreas fails to maintain this balance, it leads to an excess of glucose in the blood. This condition is called hyperglycaemia and the lack of the necessary balancing insulin is called Diabetes Mellitus which is classed as a primary condition.

There is no known clinical cause that is precise. In general terms, the cause can be hereditary, environmental or hormonal or some combination of the latter two. These include the probable cause of 'primary' diabetes that is divided further into Type I - juvenile onset, or Type II - late or maturity onset.

The cause of other forms of diabetes is known, although they are classified as secondary diabetes. These are:

- surgery
- disease   } Destruction of Islets of Langerhans &
- drugs   hormonal imbalance (secondary diabetes)
- auto-immunity

The inability of the tissues to utilise glucose, or to store it, leads to the liver attempting to redress the balance by producing sugar (glucose). It does this by converting amino acids which, in turn, interferes with the liver's fat and sugar metabolism. This causes lack of energy, apathy, mood swings, thirst and can be accompanied by weight-loss.

Other common symptoms can include blurring of vision, cramp in muscles, pruritus vulvae (itching, inflammation) and susceptibility to infection. The urine contains sugar and acetone, with a tendency to keto acidosis and high blood glucose.

The tribules of the kidneys are unable to absorb the excess level of under utilised glucose and the excess is excreted in the urine (glycosuria) which has an odour of acetone or pear drops. The patient's breadth would have the same smell of pear drops.

Remember that if a diabetic patient has not eaten recently and their blood sugar falls, they may behave as if drunk before falling into a diabetic coma. There have been incidents in which the Police have mistaken a low blood sugar diabetic as a drunk and locked them in a cell - occasionally with serious consequences. Complementary therapists should guard against making a similar mistake by being aware of the similarity of these symptoms.

The condition can be stabilised by direct intravenous injection of a balancing quantity of insulin, at prescribed intervals. For mild forms of diabetes, diet or diet plus hypoglycaemic tablets can control the condition: personal determination and discipline plays a large part for these patients.

Within the limit of our present understanding of the condition and the treatment available, the patient will have diabetes for life. They learn to adjust their diet and to self-administer insulin and this enables them to live a normal life.

A personal curiosity, however, is what causes the pancreas to malfunction originally? Particularly, in the case of late onset diabetes where the pancreas has functioned perfectly normally for many years. We can treat the symptoms and alleviate the adverse effects of the condition but, as yet, we cannot identify the root cause. One theory is that severe emotional shock can trigger the imbalance.

Chapter VII

A Few Words About Footwear

We would not wear wellies for a waltz or stilettos for a sandy beach.

Obviously, common sense avoids this light-hearted extreme and the task of finding shoes that fit and maintain the health and mobility of our feet is one of individual choice.

One simple piece of advice is to make sure that you always buy your shoes in the afternoon, when the feet are warm and have swelled a little. Also, get the assistant to check the fit while you are standing so that the foot/shoe is assessed under full body weight.

Probably, many of us are guilty of giving insufficient time and thought to the importance of a well-fitted shoe. Out of sight, out of mind applies. Men can be too impatient; women can be slaves of fashion.

Sizing can be confusing and the subject of much conjecture. At best, they serve as a guide to an initial range of choice and consequent help to the shop assistant. They may be kept fit by shinning up and down their shelf-ladder like a demented budgie but there comes a point when fitness exceeds temper! So it is wise to have some idea of our shoe-size.

Remember, that just because we were once size 9 with a medium breadth shoe when in our teens or twenties, it does not follow that this continues throughout life. Feet have a habit of spreading as we spread with age.

We buy shoes not only to fit our feet but also to fit our activity. Everyday shoes are what we wear most of the time, whereas, golf, running or football footwear are specific to their respective activity.

What to look for to achieve quality fitting

Quality of manufacture is more important than price. It is possible that a 'cheap' shoe will fit your foot better than a 'quality' brand-name shoe. That said, the following may prove useful:

Length: Make sure that the shoe is approximately ¼" longer than your longest toe (for some people their second toe is longer than their hallux, big toe). This of course refers to overall length from the back of the shoe to the front.

It is equally important to get the heel-to-ball fitting to match. This is the distance from the heel to the ball (metatarsal heads) of the foot. Shoes are designed to bend at a particular place and if the foot wants to bend naturally at a different place, there would be trouble.

Breadth: One of the most important fits to have correct, is the breadth of the shoe coincident with the forward aspect of the metatarsal heads of the foot (Figures 24 & 25). This dimension should be snug whilst allowing the toes to spread naturally under full body weight, i.e. when standing, walking or running.

Out of interest, examine your existing shoes. Hold one in front of you at eye-level and look to see if the upper has bulged over the sole - towards the very edge of the sole. If it has, the shoe is too narrow; the upper has been stretched and forced sideways to accommodate your foot (Figure 25).

<u>Depth</u>: This is not measured in the shop - unless it has an X-ray machine and even then you may not wish to be exposed to it. So it is a matter of judgement. On trying the shoe, there should be no feeling of downward pressure of the upper upon the toes. In addition, there should be a one or two degree up-slope to the toe of the shoe, as shown in Figure 24.

<u>Soles</u> need to be long-wearing, flexible and not too heavy - a bit like us! Synthetic soles often meet these criteria but these materials are not necessarily healthy for all feet.

<u>Toe Box</u> should meet the requirements of depth as mentioned earlier and be rounded not flat. Otherwise, painful, bruised nails and corns can occur.

<u>Tongue</u> should be padded, or soft leather and stitched so as to remain central to the shoe at all times.

<u>Heel Counter</u> should be a snug fit with the heel of the foot and sufficiently high to give comfortable support without cutting into or restricting the movement of the Achilles tendon.

<u>Materials</u> Leather is the favoured material for soles and for uppers because it 'breathes' and it moulds well over a last. So for those who have feet that perspire, leather is advisable because it can absorb a certain amount of moisture. When the shoes are not in use they should be left to air, preferably, with a set of shoe-trees inserted, so that the shoes keep their shape. For those with dry feet, however, synthetic materials can be chosen.

Laces versus Slip-ons

A chiropodist would prefer to see you wearing a lace-up shoe because only lacing the shoe to the foot can guarantee a snug or proper fit at the important areas of metatarsal heads, around the instep and around the ankle just below (inferior to) it (Figure 24).

A slip-on shoe is more capable of becoming a slip-off shoe. Unless it is a tight fit, the bending action of the foot, combined with toeing off, will gradually stretch the upper to a point when it cannot continue to contain the foot. A compromise - if you must have a slip-on shoe - is to buy shoes with an elasticated arch that fits just over and around the instep.

Footwear for sports people

To avoid running injuries - such as those illustrated in Figure 23 - a well-made and well designed shoe is essential. There is a bewildering choice of shapes and textures that prevent a detailed consideration. It would need a separate book. However, a few key features apply generally.

The support provided by the heel counter must not be so high as to restrict the natural sliding action of the Achilles tendon or to rub the heel above the heel bone (calcaneum).

Rounded and flared heels are most suitable for running. A bevelled heel allows the foot to 'roll' into the flat position without putting too much strain on the Achilles tendon or on the front leg muscles, e.g. anterior tibialis muscle.

Flared heels help to stabilise the foot and to avoid turning the ankle over outwards (eversion - see Figure 8) or turning the joint over inwards (inversion - see Figure 8). But flared heeled shoes or boots must never be worn for activities that require quick changes of direction - like tennis, squash or hockey. The flare then would be a serious handicap because of its quality of preventing sideways roll.   Consequently, the ankle

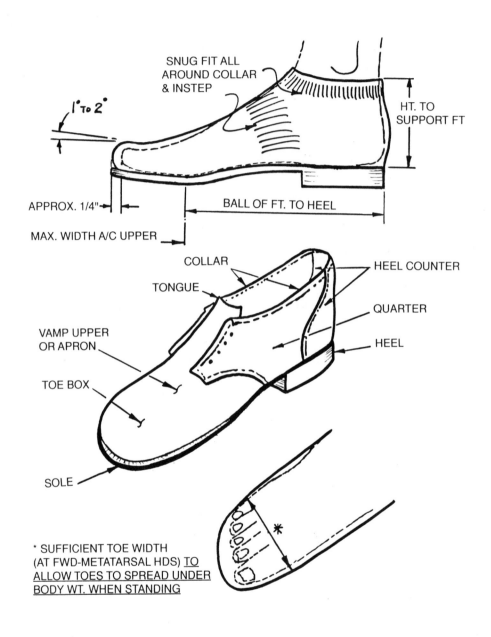

SNUG FIT ALL
AROUND COLLAR
& INSTEP

HT. TO
SUPPORT FT

1° TO 2°

APPROX. 1/4"

BALL OF FT. TO HEEL

MAX. WIDTH A/C UPPER

COLLAR

TONGUE

HEEL COUNTER

QUARTER

VAMP UPPER
OR APRON

HEEL

TOE BOX

SOLE

* SUFFICIENT TOE WIDTH
(AT FWD-METATARSAL HDS) <u>TO</u>
<u>ALLOW TOES TO SPREAD UNDER</u>
<u>BODY WT. WHEN STANDING</u>

<u>FIG 24: 'STAR QUALITY' FITTING</u>

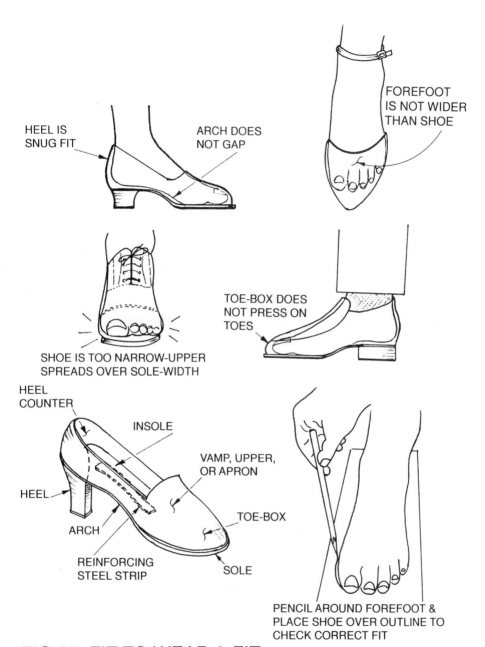

HEEL IS
SNUG FIT

ARCH DOES
NOT GAP

FOREFOOT
IS NOT WIDER
THAN SHOE

SHOE IS TOO NARROW-UPPER
SPREADS OVER SOLE-WIDTH

TOE-BOX DOES
NOT PRESS ON
TOES

HEEL
COUNTER

INSOLE

VAMP, UPPER,
OR APRON

HEEL

TOE-BOX

ARCH

REINFORCING
STEEL STRIP

SOLE

PENCIL AROUND FOREFOOT &
PLACE SHOE OVER OUTLINE TO
CHECK CORRECT FIT

FIG 25: FIT TO WEAR & FIT FOR COMFORT

would twist resulting in sprained or torn ligaments - the 'elastic bandages' that hold the ankle joint in place (Figure 6).

When you have found the style that suits you, stay with it and buy a second pair and run them in <u>before</u> your existing pair has worn out. There is good reason for alternating two pairs of running shoes. As you wear down the heel and alter the shape of the uppers, your muscle action and running pattern will be affected slightly to compensate for these differences. So if a completely new pair of shoes is worn for hard exercise without first running them in, there is a danger of pulling a muscle or risking a stress fracture.

Laces should extend down and over the instep area and thus give sufficient snug support to prevent the foot sliding backwards or forwards even when running long distances.

The tongue should be well padded to protect the instep. Look for shoes that have a sole capable of absorbing the pounding and repeated heel-strikes associated with distance running or long-jump sprints and take-offs.

If soccer, rugby or hockey is your sport the studs should be long enough to give good grip on any ground conditions. When playing or training on astro turf, soft studs or pimpled soles are suitable because on the harder surface, a certain amount of 'give' is needed.

Also, pay attention to the part of the shoe - both sole and upper - where your foot needs to bend to get maximum push off in the running gait. This area of the shoe should be flexible to allow all the toes to push off the running surface with maximum effect.

Look for a soft layer of material between the sole and the heel counter. This absorbs the shock of heel-strikes and saves the runner getting bruised heels. A cushioned sole also lessons the shock load into the lower limbs and, ultimately, into the spine.

Qualified reflexologists know the value of healthy feet and the proven relationship to constitutional health. An athlete with well designed, well fitted and purpose made shoes is not only looking after his feet, he is also looking after his general health and increasing the chances of success.

TYPES OF SHOES & BOOTS

Balmoral	Heavy walking boot	**Moccasin**	Soft, heel-less, slip-on shoe with a stitched upper
Brogan	Ankle-high work shoe	**Mukluk**	Eskimo boot of soft reindeer skin or sealskin
Brogue	Stout walking shoe with decorative punch-marks	**Mule**	Loose, backless, strapless slipper
Buckskin	Shoe made from deerskin or sheepskin	**Oxford**	Stout shoe with a low heel
Buskin, Cothurnus/ cothurn	Thick-soled, calf-length or knee-length boot, as worn by ancient Greek actors	**Pantoffle**	Slipper
Chappal	Indian leather sandal	**Patten**	Wooden overshoe or clog on a raised wooden sole or metal platform
Chukka	Suede ankle-boot, usually with two eyelets	**Peeptoe**	Shoe with the toe cut away
Court shoe	Woman's plain high-heeled shoe without fastenings	**Plimsoll, dap, gymshoe, tacky**	Light rubber-soled shoe with a cloth upper, usually laced
Espadrille	Rope-soled shoe with canvas or fabric upper	**Pump**	Light, flat or low-heeled shoe, without fastenings, often worn for dancing
Galosh	Waterproof overshoe	**Sabot**	Clog, made from a single piece of wood
Geta	Japanese wooden-soled sandal	**Sneaker**	Soft-soled shoe
Ghillie	Shoe with fringed laces	**Stiletto**	Woman's shoe with a narrow, tapering high heel
Gumshoe	Rubber shoe or overshoe; sneaker	**Velskoen/ veldskoen**	South African shoe or boot of untanned hide
Hessian boot	High, tasselled man's boot	**Wader**	Very high waterproof boot, as worn by anglers
Larrigan	Moccasin with knee-length leggings	**Wellington**	Unlaced rubber boot for wet conditions; high leather riding boot
Loafer	Casual shoe resembling a moccasin	**Winkle-picker**	Man's shoe with a very pointed toe

Reproduced by kind permission of Reader's Digest.

FURTHER READING

'Physical Examination of the Spine & Extremities'
by Stanley Hoppenfeld.
Pub. Appleton - Century - Crofts, ISBN 0-8385-7853-5,
ref. Chapter 8 of an extremely well illustrated book.

'Common Foot Disorders' by Donald Neale, OBE
and Isobel Adams.
Churchill Livingstone, ISBN 0-443-03285-8.

'Foot & Ankle Pain' by Rene Cailliet, MD.
Cailliet F.A. Davis, ISBN - 0-8036-1601-5.

'A Colour Atlas of Foot & Ankle Anatomy'
by R.M.H. McMinn, R.T. Hutchings & B.M. Logan,
Wolfe Medical Publications Ltd., ISBN - 0-7234-0782-7.

'A Colour Atlas of the Nail in Clinical Diagnosis'
by D.W. Beaven & S.E. Brooks.
Wolfe Medical Publications Ltd., ISBN - 0-7234-0826-2.

USEFUL ADDRESSES

*The SMAE Institute & The British Chriopody
& Podiatry Association*
149 Bath Road,
The New Hall,
Maidenhead,
SL6 4LA
U.K.

The International Institute of Reflexology®
Head Office   UK Head Office
P.O. Box 12642   255 Turleigh
St. Petersburg   Bradford-on-Avon
Florida 33733-2642   Wiltshire
U.S.A.   BA15 2HG
                               U.K.

The Association of Reflexologists
Katepwa House
Ashfield Park Avenue
Ross-on-Wye
Herefordshire
HR9 5AX
U.K.

The Northern Institute of Massage
14-16 St. Mary's Place
Bury
Lancashire
BL9 0DZ
U.K.

INDEX

D

E

F

M

N

O

S

Synthetic soles 77

NOTES

NOTES